PREGNANCY

EXPECTING A BABY FOR FIRST TIME MOMS

A COMPLETE PREGNANCY GUIDE

FOR NEW PARENTS

BY HELEN WHITE

Disclaimer

TABLE OF CONTENTS

INTRODUCTION

Thank you for purchasing "Pregnancy: Expecting A Baby for First Time Moms: A Complete Pregnancy Guide for New Parents". As well, congratulations on your pregnancy! This precious time in life is one of the most emotional, challenging, and rewarding times in your entire life. You should expect for things to be very different during this time, as you are undergoing a number of changes in your life that are nothing like what you would expect. However, this transitional period is an excellent opportunity to prepare yourself for what's yet to come: emotionally, mentally, spiritually, and physically.

Becoming a new parent is an exciting experience, whether your pregnancy was expected or unexpected. You may not always feel that pregnancy glow that people rave about, but you can certainly do things to help the experience feel amazing overall. In this book, you are going to learn about exactly what to expect, and how you can make pregnancy as peaceful and enjoyable as possible.

You should remember that pregnancy, labor, and parenthood experiences are going to be different from person to person. No family will experience this journey the same, and so you should prepare to have your own unique experiences along the way. While you can certainly receive guidance and support from others, you should take the time to acknowledge that you are not going to experience things the exact same as everyone else. At this time, you should give yourself permission to experience pregnancy, labor and parenthood in the way that suits you, perfectly. The sooner you allow yourself the chance to experience your unique journey uniquely, the more positive your experience will be overall.

This pregnancy guidebook has been carefully designed to allow you the opportunity to make this journey as comfortable and enjoyable as possible for you. Inside, you will learn all about what to expect during each trimester, including that fourth trimester that people don't talk about often enough. You will also have the opportunity to explore some helpful tips based on your unique family dynamics. As well, if there is a father or a partner present in your journey, a special section has been created just for them, so they can help you through this precious time in your life, too! Each chapter has been thoughtfully designed to help you achieve maximum knowledge on this time in your life, and how you can make the most out of it. Please remember that if something doesn't apply to your unique situation, you do not need to worry about it. If you're ready to learn all about pregnancy and this exciting journey, please dive on in, and remember: enjoy!

CHAPTER ONE: WHAT TO EXPECT IN YOUR FIRST TRIMESTER

The first trimester is an exciting, emotional, and taxing time for virtually everyone who becomes pregnant. During this time, you may feel a number of different emotions and symptoms as you mentally and physically prepare to embrace the coming months, and years. Some women report this to be the easiest trimester, and others report it to be the worst. How you will experience it in your own journey will depend on many factors that are beyond your control. However, you can brace yourself for certain experiences and equip yourself with knowledge on how to make this first stretch of your journey as comfortable as possible.

SYMPTOMS AND DIFFICULTIES

The first trimester comes with a significant number of new symptoms and experiences, since it is the first leg of your entire pregnancy! At this time, you are going to experience things you have likely never felt before, and it can be difficult for some women. For some, there are minimal symptoms during this part of your journey. Others seem to experience every single symptom possible, and it can be very difficult to endure, both physically and emotionally. Below is a list of symptoms you might experience, and some things you can do to help make it as comfortable as possible for you.

MISSED PERIOD

While this isn't always the first symptom for pregnant women, it is a sure-fire way to start expecting that something is up. If you miss your period, you can probably guess that you are pregnant. You can either take a home pregnancy test, and then book an appointment with your doctor, or simply go straight to booking an appointment. Many women prefer to test from home for a quick answer to the ultimate question: "am I pregnant?" Others prefer to wait until their doctors' appointment. Your doctor will test to confirm your pregnancy, so it is not a big deal if you don't test from home beforehand.

MORNING SICKNESS

Many women are familiar with this symptom, whether they've been pregnant before or not. Morning sickness is a symptom that is commonly talked about in movies, talk shows, and virtually anywhere that pregnancy is being talked about. When people are pregnant, the most common symptom they'll experience before others is nausea. Not every woman will experience morning sickness, but many will. Morning sickness is not restricted to the morning, either. In fact, you can experience this symptom at any time during the day, and even multiple times during the day. The best way to combat morning sickness is to eat several small meals throughout the day, since it seems to be triggered by an empty stomach. You can also focus on eating starchy foods, such as mashed potatoes, crackers, breads, and others that will help keep your tummy full and absorb the stomach acid. As well, many report that ginger is great with this symptom. You can eat candied ginger, make a ginger tea, or consume it in any other way that works for you. Another method you may find that works is to take a Vitamin B6 supplement. You should ask your doctor before beginning any supplements, especially during pregnancy, but if you are really struggling, this may help. Finally, if you are one of the unlucky women who is sick to no end, and can't seem to find anything natural to help you, you should talk to your doctor about your morning sickness. In some cases, they may provide you with a medicine you can take to help alleviate the symptoms and make it easier for you to get all of the important nutrients and stay hydrated during this precious time in your journey!

FOOD CRAVINGS AND AVERSIONS

This symptom can be closely linked with morning sickness. Some women find that certain foods will trigger their sickness to be worse, so if that's what you're experiencing, feel free to eliminate those foods from your diet for now! Food cravings are one of the most commonly talked about symptoms as well, but food aversions, not so much! When you are pregnant, you might start to experience sudden and strong cravings for random foods, even ones that normally don't go well together. You may also develop strong aversions to foods, with certain tastes, textures, or smells of food turning you away from being hungry, or making you feel ill altogether!

If you are experiencing cravings, you are generally safe to indulge in these cravings. Just make sure that you aren't eating excessive amounts of sugars or other unhealthy food items, to avoid dealing with complications later in pregnancy!

If you are experiencing aversions, you should look for other ways to supplement your diet with things you may not be getting enough of. For example, if you are turned off of milk, you can try getting your calcium intake through low-fat cheese, yogurt, or even cottage cheese. If these ingredients alone are still upsetting to you, you can try adding them into a recipe such as with a sauce or a soup to help you get your calcium in. Or, if you are turned off of meat, you can try alternative protein sources like beans. Ultimately, there are many ways to make sure you are getting your proper food intake. Just make sure you are getting your proper nutritional intake! You can speak with your doctor for more ideas on alternatives, if you need to.

SENSE OF SMELL

During pregnancy, many women report having a stronger sense of smell. One theory of this symptom is that this could assist you in avoiding foods that may be particularly dangerous to you during pregnancy. If you are experiencing a heightened sense of smell, you may choose to keep yourself surrounded by smells that are less repulsive to you. A great way to combat your sense of smell if you are struggling with a smell that is repulsive to you is to keep a favorite body spray and piece of cloth handy, and lightly spray the cloth and keep it in your vicinity so it keeps the air around you smelling pleasant. This can greatly help with anyone who feels that their sense of smell is contributing to their food aversions or morning sickness.

FATIGUE

The first trimester of pregnancy can be one of the hardest for fatigue. You may feel like all you want to do is nap, and you should know that this is completely normal. There are a few things that contribute to this symptom. First, this symptom can be from all of the extra work your body is putting in to growing another human being. It takes a lot of energy for your body to do all of the extra work! Second, this symptom can be related to the hormone progesterone, which can have a sedative effect on your body. For some women, excessive fatigue may be related to anemia which can be caused by a slight iron deficiency due to your body having to produce an additional 50% blood volume for the growing fetus. If you are experiencing this, your doctor will find it in your initial blood screening, and will help you level out the problem through iron pills. If you get your blood test done, and your doctor does not feel that anemia is an issue for you, you don't need to worry about this.

There are three primary ways to combat the tiredness you may experience in your first trimester. First, you can get moving. A slight stretch or a short walk around the block can greatly help you wake up if you are struggling to stay awake. Keeping yourself busy and moving from one task to the next is a great way to keep yourself from becoming or staying excessively tired. Another way is to take your prenatal vitamins. They contain enough nutrients to help keep your levels up and prevent anemia or other energy-deficiencies that could be related to a lower food intake. Finally, you should sleep whenever you can. Going to bed earlier, napping when you can, and relaxing whenever possible is a great way to help nurture your body through this exhausting time. If you are feeling particularly tired and simply can't push through it, don't over exert your body. Take it as a cue, and go to sleep.

FREQUENT URINATION

This is another famous symptom of pregnancy, and believe it or not, it starts as early as the first trimester! Many people believe this symptom is caused by the baby pressing on your bladder, but you can start experiencing it within' the first few weeks of your pregnancy, too! In fact, most women do! This is caused by your kidneys working overtime to flush out any toxins from your body, as well as from your growing uterus: which is actually growing faster than you might think! Despite needing to pee a significant amount, you should absolutely not decrease your fluid intake. As well, don't hold it if you have to go, as this can cause an infection! The best thing to do is urinate when you need to, and reduce caffeine intake, such as through coffee, because it is a bladder stimulant! (As well, too much caffeine isn't good for your growing baby!) When you go to the bathroom, you can always lean forward after you feel you are done, to help make sure you get rid of everything in your bladder. This will help you completely empty your bladder every time, hopefully helping prevent you from having to go quite as often.

ACNE

This is another symptom that can be blamed on pregnancy hormones. Not everyone experiences that beautiful pregnancy glow, especially in the first trimester. For some women, this symptom eases up in the second trimester, but for others it maintains itself all the way through pregnancy and even for some time after. The best way to combat this symptom is to gently clean your skin on a regular basis. Make sure you don't over-wash or over-scrub as you can further aggravate or even damage your delicate facial skin, but make sure you are washing it on a regular basis. You can also try switching to a gentler face wash and a moisturizer that is oil-free, to help prevent it from further clogging your pores. Finally, make sure your skin care products don't contain harsh acne treating chemicals like salicylic acid, retinols, steroids, or benzoyl peroxides. These have been linked to birth defects, so it is a good idea to refrain from using them. Try something more gentle, such as a face wash with charcoal in it, which is a great natural acne-treating cleaner.

BREATHLESSNESS

Even though you don't have a baby pressing on your lungs just yet, you can still experience breathlessness! You can chalk this one up to hormones, as well. This happens because your body requires more oxygen to satisfy all of the extra blood in your body. So, even though you might be getting tons of oxygen into your lungs, you might feel like you are not getting enough. This is completely normal. Take it easy, don't over exert yourself, and sit down when you need to!

HEADACHES

Another symptom of pregnancy is headaches. These are especially common during the first trimester. They are usually caused by low blood sugar, which is a symptom of your changing metabolism, or from an increase in hormones. In order to help eliminate the symptoms of your headache, you can use hot or cold compresses, get some fresh air, or massage your temples. If these don't work, you can try taking Children's Tylenol. You may also speak with your doctor for assistance with relieving these symptoms.

CHANGES IN VISION

A symptom that a lot of people don't talk about includes changes in vision that can occur during pregnancy. This is caused by having an increase in your blood flow. What happens is everything in your body swells up a little, including your eyes. This can cause your cornea to thicken and curve more, which can cause changes in your vision. For those who wear contacts, you may have to switch to wearing glasses until your pregnancy ends. If you don't experience changes in vision, you may experience excessively dry eyes. The best way to combat this symptom is to use eye drops to lubricate your eyes and keep them from drying out.

Swollen Breasts

Your breasts start getting ready to nurse your new baby as soon as you become pregnant! Even though your baby is still tiny, and doesn't even resemble a human yet, your breasts are already getting ready to give your baby milk! Hormonal changes are responsible for this happening so rapidly. If you are experiencing swollen breasts, and if this symptom is painful or uncomfortable for you, there are a few things you can do to combat these. First, you can buy larger bras that have extra rows of hooks to make easy adjustments as you go. You should avoid bras that are front closing, as these can create more pain for those who are experiencing tenderness. You can also invest in a cotton sports-style bra to sleep in, which will prevent soreness if you are experiencing it during your sleep.

CHANGES IN LIBIDO

Your change in libido can go one of two ways. During pregnancy, a larger amount of blood flows to your vagina and clitoris, making them extremely sensitive. For some women, this makes sex even more enjoyable, and they find that they may be turned in an excessive amount. Simple things such as changing underwear or sitting on a different textured surface can trigger you to become turned on. For other women, it is the complete opposite, and the idea of sex may be a complete turn off. Whatever end of the spectrum you are on is completely normal, and you should honor that in yourself. As well, make sure you maintain open communication with your partner, so he or she does not begin to feel insecure or rejected by your change in libido. If you are not feeling sexual, you may wish to keep your intimacy up in more appealing ways, such as back rubs, cuddles, and holding hands.

EMOTIONAL CHANGES

Many things play into the emotional changes you may experience during pregnancy. Lack of sleep, changes in hormones, and even the idea of pregnancy itself can all contribute to the emotions you may experience when you are pregnant. These may be a little more pressing in the first trimester than they will be later on, once the reality of your pregnancy becomes more comfortable to you, and your body begins to adjust to the changes in hormones. If you find that you are experiencing emotions in a more extreme way, or if you feel that you are rapidly switching between emotions, you should know it is completely normal. The best thing you can do is rest up, and get exercise, as these will help balance out your emotions as much as possible by alleviating stress. As well, you can seek support in friends, family and professionals both on and offline in order to help keep your support system strong and contribute to your emotional and mental comfort during this time.

Doctors' Appointments and Medical Tests

There are a few doctors' appointments you will attend during your first trimester of pregnancy. During this trimester, your doctor will likely want to see you on a monthly basis. This is a chance for your doctor to keep their file updated on your medical profile during pregnancy, and detect any challenges that arise, or assist you in preventing them altogether.

Your very first doctors visit should be booked when you miss your period, or otherwise think you may be pregnant. At this time, your doctor is going to want to check to confirm your pregnancy. You will likely take a urine test at the time of the doctors' appointment, and then they will request that you get a blood sample taken to confirm your pregnancy. This blood test also helps your doctor detect any issues that may be present, such as anemia or blood sugar-related issues. They will also book your first ultrasound or sonogram, which will take place between 12 and 14 weeks. This is also known as the dating ultrasound, which will help your doctor create a more accurate due date for your pregnancy.

After your first doctors' appointment, the succeeding ones in your first trimester will be relatively simple. Each time you attend an appointment, your doctor will check a few things to keep track of yours and your baby's health during your pregnancy. He or she will check your blood pressure and your pulse. They will also require that you provide a urine sample at each visit, which allows them to measure your ketones to ensure your organs are functioning effectively during pregnancy. After that, your doctor will check your baby's heart rate. Finally, they will ask you if you have any questions, and check to make sure your symptoms are normal and that you are coping well with all of the changes. At these appointments, you may wish to bring your partner, a trusted friend or family member, or your labor coach if you have chosen to hire one. It is a good idea for these individuals to join you, if they will be a part of your pregnancy and labor experience, because it will give them the opportunity to help support you more effectively.

If you have any questions during your pregnancy, you should keep track of them in a diary or a note book. This will help make sure you get all of your questions answered when you attend doctors' visits. The infamous "Mommy brain" starts as early as your first trimester, which means it can be harder for you to remember things. This is why it is important that you write things down that you may wish to ask your doctor, or that you feel may be important for your doctor to know about.

During your pregnancy, if you ever experience something that seems abnormal, such as bleeding, excessive cramping, or severe symptoms that are difficult to manage on your own, it is important that you contact your doctor. You should not wait until your next appointment to discuss this issues. Instead, you should book an appointment for as soon as possible. If you feel the symptoms are an emergency, you should not hesitate to attend your local hospital and seek assistance. During pregnancy, you will be cared for by the maternity ward of your hospital, as they are better capable of providing you care that will keep you and your fetus as healthy as possible.

CONCLUSION

The first trimester of pregnancy can be taxing: physically, emotionally, and mentally. During this time, you may feel a number of different emotions and symptoms that could make it hard for you to feel comfortable or truly enjoy your pregnancy. There are several things you can do to help yourself through this time, and you should do your best to keep your comfort levels a priority.

Make sure you are staying healthy and active, which you can learn more about in Chapter 4 of this guide. As well, you should prepare for your doctors' appointments, and make sure you are telling them everything you feel they need to know. As much as you can, you should relax and nurture your body through the first trimester, so it is more capable of handling all of the added stresses that pregnancy can bring about.

Chapter Two: What to Expect in Your Second Trimester

The second trimester tends to be a lot easier for some women, but for others it can continue to be difficult. As with all other experiences during pregnancy, it can be hard to predict which it will be for you. There are different symptoms you are likely to experience at this time, each of which also has its own set of recommended "treatments". This trimester lasts from week 13 to week 27, making it the longest trimester of your entire pregnancy.

Symptoms and Difficulties

The symptoms you experience during the second trimester will likely be different from those you experienced in the first trimester. For the second trimester, you will continue to experience a lot of the symptoms you had in the first trimester. However, you may notice that your headaches, morning sickness, and excessive fatigue settle down during these weeks. The additional symptoms you may experience include the following ones listed below.

Dry or Itchy Skin

Many women experience dry or itchy skin in their second trimester. This is usually experienced most in the belly area, and is likely due to the stretching of the skin at a rapid rate.

You may start to get stretch marks, as well as feel really dry and itchy. You can combat these symptoms by using gentle lotions on your tummy. There are even some that are specially made for stretchmark prevention, which you may choose to use to keep the skin hydrated and prevent yourself from getting an excessive number of stretchmarks. You should note, however, that these are not always effective in preventing stretchmarks, and you will likely still experience them.

CHANGED LIBIDO

Your sex drive is still going to be significantly different at this point. For most women, the second trimester is when their libido will come back, if they ever lost it. This will make having sex more pleasurable for them, and potentially even increase their desire to have sex. During pregnancy, it is completely safe to have sex, unless your doctor says otherwise. However, as your tummy continues to grow, you will want to prevent laying on your back or your stomach for sex. Laying on your side, going on your hands and knees, or using pillows to support your body are all great ways to make it more comfortable and prevent yourself from putting excessive pressure on your uterus. Additionally, you will want to be very open when communicating with your partner, to ensure they don't do anything that will be painful or uncomfortable for you. If you continue to feel as though you don't desire to have sex, you should not feel pressured to have sex. Go with what your body tells you, and you will be fine.

LEG PAINS

Stretching ligaments, hormones, change in gravity center, and added weight all contribute to leg pains you may experience during pregnancy. You might notice that when you are sleeping (or trying to) you experience leg cramping. This type of cramping can be caused by pressure being put on nerves in your body. Try adjusting your sleeping position and using body pillows and other pillows to give your growing belly more support and take some of the pressure off of your back and hips. If this is happening during the day, try and reduce the amount of time you spend on your feet, invest in high quality shoes with comfortable insoles, and do your best to maintain a healthy posture during pregnancy.

PUFFINESS

Due to the increased blood flow in your body, you may notice that even your ankles, wrists, hands, and face will begin to swell during the second trimester. This is totally normal, and occurs because your blood circulation will be slower, and your body will be holding on to more fluids than normal. If you feel that your legs, ankles or feet are swelling excessively, or you feel that you are getting faint or light headed often, you should consider discussing this with your doctor, as it could be related to a low blood pressure.

ACHES

Just like you are more likely to experience leg pains, you are also more likely to experience back, hip, shoulder, and pelvic pain when you are in your second trimester. This is for all of the same reasons as you may experience leg pains and cramping. Your pregnancy hormones will be relaxing the ligaments which means your bones will be starting to adjust in order to prepare for labor. The best thing you can do is keep your posture as healthy as possible, stay off of your feet when you can, and avoid from over exerting yourself. If you feel uncomfortable or like you need a rest, stop what you are doing and focus on getting comfortable for a few minutes to help eliminate the aches.

ABDOMINAL PAIN AND STRETCHING

As the ligaments loosen and stretch, and your belly continues to grow, you may notice more pain in your abdominal area. The skin and muscles could feel raw and painful due to all of the rapid growth, which is completely normal. The best thing you can do is keep this area hydrated with lotion, and use warm compresses on the painful areas to help alleviate the pain and make it a little more comfortable for yourself. Unfortunately, you will not likely be able to prevent or eliminate this feeling completely.

Loose Teeth

Because the ligaments and bones in your body are being loosened due to pregnancy hormones, you may also discover that your teeth become loose during pregnancy. This should go away after pregnancy, so try to keep yourself from playing with these loose teeth and do your best to ignore them. If you notice excessive bleeding or swelling in your gums, you should seek treatment as these can be a sign of periodontal disease, which is something you don't want to experience, particularly during pregnancy. Light bleeding, particularly during brushing, is generally not a big deal, though. This is common due to the increased blood volume in your body.

Nasal Discomforts

Another symptom of increased blood volume is nasal congestion, and nosebleeds. If you notice you are starting to get nosebleeds or that you are constantly congested, it is likely due to your pregnancy hormones. Unless you have major nosebleeds that are causing symptoms like lightheadedness, you should be okay. Still, this is a good thing to discuss with your doctor, so they can keep record of it and ensure that it does not become an issue for you during your pregnancy.

Heart Burns

This classic pregnancy symptom is an uncomfortable one that can be hard to manage. This is caused by your growing uterus putting pressure on your stomach, forcing food and stomach acids back up into your esophagus, which can cause the burning sensation. You can eliminate this by eating smaller meals, nibbling on starchy snacks like saltines, or drinking a small amount of milk. If you are experiencing excessive heartburn that is causing significant discomfort, you may consider bringing this up with your doctor, who may be able to recommend a pregnancy-safe antacid for you to use.

URINARY TRACT INFECTIONS

Due to increased frequency in urination and a more frequently filled bladder, you may notice that you get increased risk towards developing urinary tract infections. You may even find that you develop a few during pregnancy. This is caused by hormonal changes that are slowing the flow of your urine, and your growing uterus stopping your bladder from emptying completely due to added pressures. If you notice any symptoms of a urinary tract infection, such as a burning sensation when you pee, an even higher number of daily urinations with decreased outflow, a strong odor or presence of blood in the urine, you should consult your doctor immediately. It is important that urinary tract infections are dealt with as soon as possible, to prevent possible complications they may cause in your pregnancy.

BRAXTON HICKS CONTRACTIONS

These can also be referred to as false labor. Braxton Hicks contractions are basically practice contractions that your uterus does while it is preparing for labor and delivery. When you are having these contractions, you may feel a very tight and hard sensation in your belly that may or may not be accompanied by a painful sensation. In order to be classified as Braxton Hicks contractions, this sensation should go away within' a few minutes and should not return in any form of a regular pattern. If you appear to be having regular and painful contractions that are persistent despite you changing your position or walking around, you should call your doctor in case you are experiencing preterm labor symptoms.

DOCTORS' APPOINTMENTS AND MEDICAL TESTS

In your second trimester, you are going to experience a lot of the same things as you did in your first trimester. Just like before, your doctor is going to want to check your urine, your blood pressure and pulse, and your baby's heartbeat. They will also measure your abdomen, check the position of your baby, and perform any other related medical tests that may be unique to your situation. For example, if you have been experiencing anemia, or symptoms of anemia, your doctor may want to check your blood levels to see if this is an issue for you.

You are also going to be asked about the symptoms you are experiencing, and you should expect for your care provider to tell you about what to expect in the coming weeks. Towards the end of your second trimester, you may start visiting your doctor every second week, instead of every month.

During your second trimester, you will have to complete a glucose test. This gives your doctors information about your blood sugar levels, and lets them know if your body is dealing with your blood sugar contents efficiently. If not, you may be experiencing prenatal diabetes, which can be managed with changes in diet and some medications. Additionally, you will have an ultrasound done around 20 weeks which will allow the doctor to ensure you are progressing normally. You may also find out the sex of your baby, if you wish to do so. Some parents even choose to get a 3D ultrasound booked with a special clinic so that they can see their baby in a 3D format.

Other tests you may be asked to do include a triple screen, which can give doctors a heads up as to whether or not your fetus is at risk for diseases such as down syndrome, trisomy 18 syndrome, or spina bifida. You may also get a cell-free fetal DNA test to check for chromosomal disorders. Finally, if your triple screen or cell-free fetal DNA tests come back with worrisome results, your doctor may ask you to do an amniocentesis test, which gives them a definitive diagnosis. These tests are generally uncommon, however, and will only be recommended if your doctor feels that your pregnancy is at-risk. The average healthy pregnant woman will not be asked to or required to take these tests. Even still, you will have the right to decline these tests should you feel the need to.

CONCLUSION

Your second trimester is going to bring about many more symptoms that you may or may not experience. These symptoms are mostly related to your growing body, and the continuous rise in your hormones. Most of them are easy to manage, and shouldn't cause you an excessive amount of discomfort. If they do, however, you should do your best to try and alleviate the symptoms as much as you can.

Make sure you continue to keep your communication open with your doctor, and ask any questions you may have. You should also notify your doctor about any worries or concerns you may have. As well, anyone who is involved in your pregnancy with you, such as a partner, friend, family member, or labor coach, should all be kept in the loop about your condition and symptoms. This will help them support you to the best of their ability.

The medical tests you will do are relatively simple, and for the most part you shouldn't have to do anything major during this trimester in the way of medical tests. The average healthy pregnancy should only require for you to do a blood glucose test, a 20-week ultrasound or sonogram, and your routine visits. Anything else would be recommended to you by your doctor, should they feel you need it.

CHAPTER THREE: WHAT TO EXPECT IN YOUR THIRD TRIMESTER

The third trimester is the final trimester of your actual pregnancy! While many believe that pregnancy will continue into a fourth trimester, or your postpartum period, your physical pregnancy will be done by the end of this trimester! That is, you will be giving birth to your baby! This final trimester brings a whole new myriad of symptoms, if you didn't already guess that, but at the same time after all of this practice, you are probably more than ready to manage them!

During the third trimester, you are going to want to be extra cautious of your body, because this is when labor will happen! For some women, labor happens on or after their due date, but for others they can go into early labor. It is important that you stay in tune with your body so you can alert your doctor if any major changes occur. In this chapter, you will learn what normal symptoms are, and what you should look out for! As well, you will learn more about what to expect with your doctors' visits.

SYMPTOMS

The symptoms you will experience in the third trimester are different, but not terribly different, from those you have already experienced. For the most part, they will simply be exaggerated versions of the symptoms you've already been experiencing. However, there are a few additional ones you might experience. You can learn all about it below!

LEG PAINS

This trimester, you are going to continue to experience the leg pains you have already likely been experiencing throughout the second trimester. The larger you get, the more pressure it puts on your legs and it can become very painful. Luckily, these will go away once your baby is born! In the meantime, you should do your best to stay off of your feet for long periods of time. You can also drink coconut milk or eat bananas, which are both rich in potassium, a nutrient that can significantly help reduce leg cramping.

NECK AND SHOULDER PAIN

Your growing belly is putting a lot of forward pressure on your back, which can also affect your neck and shoulders. You may notice your neck and shoulders are feeling just as bad as your lower back feels. This is completely normal. The best thing you can do is take a warm bath (but not hot!), get gentle massages, and relax a lot. If you find that it is affecting your sleep, try using body pillows and other pillows to help you support your back, legs, and belly.

HUNGRY, BUT NOT

A symptom many women report feeling that is extremely uncomfortable is the feeling that they are incredibly hungry, but are not able to eat. This is because your body needs more nutrition in order to support the growing baby. However, because your baby is getting so big, your stomach is running out of room! That means you don't have to eat as much to feel incredibly full. The best way to combat this symptom is to eat high-protein and nutrient rich mini-meals several times throughout the day. This will help keep you full and give your body all of the nutrients it needs without feeling excessively full.

LACK OF BLADDER CONTROL

Many people experience lack of bladder control when they are in their late pregnancy stages. The best thing to do is stay near a washroom, and relieve your bladder regularly. You may also wish to wear a pad if you will be going out, as they help to keep you from accidentally peeing your pants. As well, you may wish to lean forward when you are peeing to help get all of the urine out of your bladder, as the pressure of your baby may prevent you from eliminating your bladder completely.

CONSTIPATION

While your urine may be hard to stop, your bowels may slow down all on their own. This is caused, again, by all of the pressures and hormones going on in your body. You can combat this symptom through eating dates, prunes, and other fiber-rich foods that can help keep things flowing. As well, make sure you're staying hydrated, as that is important for you and your body, and it will help keep things moving.

DOCTOR VISITS AND MEDICAL TESTS

Your third trimester is going to be the most intensive one you will experience in regards to doctors' appointments. Towards the end of your third trimester, you are going to have your doctor visits increase to weekly visits. The exact time this will happen will depend on your doctor, the healthiness of your pregnancy, and whether or not you have been showing any signs of labor.

The doctors' appointments in this trimester will continue to include all of the same things as previous ones did: they will weigh you, measure your abdomen, check your blood pressure and pulse, and take a urine sample to check for protein in the urine. Towards the end of the trimester, you will likely also get pelvic exams to see if your cervix is dilating at all. At the end of each appointment, you will be informed of what to look for in the coming days.

You actually won't experience any medical examinations this trimester, unless you are carrying an at-risk pregnancy. If you have high or low blood pressure, gestational diabetes, or any other pregnancy ailment, your doctor may require you to get an ultrasound or blood test taken to monitor your pregnancy a little more closely. Otherwise, you will not experience any further medical tests!

CHAPTER FOUR: PREGNANCY SYMPTOMS YOU SHOULD NOT IGNORE

For many women, the third trimester goes all the way through effortlessly. For others, particularly those who are carrying at-risk pregnancies, you might run into a few complications. While your doctor has likely discussed this with you, particularly if you are known to be a high risk pregnancy, it can still be good to have this knowledge on hand. The following symptoms are things you should never avoid during your pregnancy. If any of these occur, you should call your doctor immediately or head to the maternity ward at your hospital.

EXCESSIVE PAIN ANYWHERE IN YOUR BELLY

Experiencing aches and pains is completely normal during pregnancy, especially in the third trimester. As your baby grows more and more, he or she will be running out of room and you may experience pain due to your baby's movement. However, if you are experiencing severe pain that is not related to the baby moving around, regardless of where it is in your stomach, you should call your doctor right away. You should be sure to monitor it especially if this pain persists or won't go away no matter what you do.

A High Fever with No Symptoms

If you have an extremely high fever but aren't experiencing symptoms of the flu, you should contact your doctor right away. This is not a common symptom late in pregnancy, and could indicate that you are presently fighting an infection. Your doctor will be able to help you confirm an accurate diagnosis and help reduce your fever depending on what he or she discovers.

Excessive Visual Disturbances

While a slight change in vision is normal during pregnancy, excessive visual disturbances are not. If you are experiencing double vision, blurred vision, dimming or flashing spots, or other lights that are lasting for more than two hours or that are making you feel unwell, you should call your doctor right away. These symptoms are not normal and should be addressed immediately.

Extreme Swelling in Hands and Feet

Swelling due to increased blood volume and fluid retention is normal, but extreme or excessive swelling in your hands and feet are not. If these symptoms appear suddenly or are accompanied by a headache or problems with your vision, you should contact your doctor.

Severe Headache that Won't Go Away

If you are experiencing a sudden and bad headache that won't go away after two to three hours, you should contact your doctor. If you are experiencing a headache alongside excessive swelling or visual disturbances, you should call your doctor right away and get seen as soon as possible.

Any Amount of Vaginal Bleeding

When labor is about to start, you may experience something called a bloody show, which we will talk more about in the next chapter. However, if you experience bleeding that is heavy, light, dark, or otherwise abnormal, you should contact your doctor. In the earlier stages of pregnancy, light spotting is usually just implantation bleeding. However, any time after implantation, any amount of blood may be a concern. You should also look out for other symptoms, such as abdominal pain or back pain, which can be a potential sign of miscarriage.

Fluids Leaking from Your Vagina

It is really common for you to experience an increase in cervical discharge, as your body is working harder to keep potential bacteria build up out of your body to prevent infections. However, if you notice a watery fluid leaking from your vagina before 37 weeks, you will need to call your doctor right away. They will likely want to admit you to the hospital to check on your membranes and make sure they haven't ruptured. If they have, they will need to treat you to help prevent infection and prepare you and your baby for a potential premature labor and birth.

A Sudden and Dramatic Increase in Thirst, With Reduced Urination

Pregnant women are at risk for dehydration, so it is important that you are drinking a lot of water throughout your entire pregnancy. However, if you notice that you are suddenly starting to feel extremely thirsty, and you aren't urinating as often, you will want to talk to your doctor. This can be a symptom of dehydration, or it can be a symptom of gestational diabetes. Your doctor is the only person who can determine the exact cause, so you will need to speak with them to get assistance.

Urinary Tract Infection Symptoms

Urinary tract infections can be particularly dangerous during pregnancy, so you will want to discuss any UTI symptoms you may experience with your doctor. They will treat you and help ensure that the infection does not affect your uterus or your growing baby.

Severe or Excessive Vomiting

Vomiting has the ability to cause dehydration and weakness in anyone, but especially a pregnant mother. While vomiting itself doesn't necessarily indicate anything is wrong, and it won't hurt your baby, you should make sure you keep your doctor in the loop about this. This will help them monitor you and ensure you aren't becoming severely dehydrated. If you are vomiting too much, you may need to be admitted to the hospital to receive fluids in order to keep you hydrated.

If you are later in your pregnancy and start suddenly vomiting an excessive amount, especially with a pain just below the ribs, you should call your doctor right away. This can be a symptom of a few different complications, all of which will need to be treated by a doctor.

FAINTING OR DIZZINESS

If you haven't eaten enough during the day, you may experience fainting or dizziness. However, it can also be caused by low blood pressure. It is important that you contact your doctor about this symptom if it is persistent, or if you faint at all. They will want to make sure that you are well, and work with you to prevent it from happening again.

SLOWED DOWN FETAL MOVEMENTS

Most often, your doctor will ask you to monitor fetal movements, to ensure your baby is moving regularly. If at any time you realize you have not felt your baby move in a while, or you perform a kick count and your baby is not as active as normal, you will want to contact your doctor. In most cases, this simply means the baby is resting. However, in some extreme cases, this can be a problem that needs to be addressed immediately.

OVERALL ITCHING, SEVERE ITCHINESS

When you are pregnant, you are likely to experience itchiness in your belly and back area as your skin stretches and grows to accommodate for the growing baby. However, if you are noticing that your entire body is extremely itchy, particularly in your palms and the soles of your feet, you should call your doctor.

SYMPTOMS OF JAUNDICE

Any symptoms of jaundice need to be immediately addressed by your doctor. This can include: yellowed skin or eyes, dark urine, and pale stools. If you have any of these symptoms, you need to talk to your doctor immediately as they will want to have you admitted to the hospital for treatment. Jaundice is caused by an underactive or infected liver, and this needs to be addressed immediately.

IF YOU FALL OR EXPERIENCE A TRAUMA TO YOUR BELLY

If at any time in your pregnancy you fall or experience some kind of trauma to your belly, such as it being hit by something, you need to visit your doctor. While your belly will be fairly resilient, it is still important that you doctor ensures nothing has impacted the baby in a bad way. You should call your doctor immediately after a fall or blow to your belly to get help.

IF SOMETHING JUST "FEELS" EXTREMELY WRONG

Some women do not have an exact symptom of anything wrong, they simply feel extremely wrong. If you think something is not right with your body, baby, or pregnancy overall, you should talk to your doctor. They will look over your vital signs and ensure everything is wrong. While in many instances this can arise from anxiety, in some cases this feeling can indicate something is wrong, despite no symptoms really being present. Always trust your intuition!

Chapter Five: Labor and Delivery

Labor and delivery carries its own set of signs and symptoms, and things you should look out for. Unlike the three trimesters of your pregnancy, these symptoms are not going to last you very long, maybe a few hours to a few days at most. Some women may experience early labor symptoms for up to a week before labor starts, but these will generally be low in intensity until they get closer to active labor.

In this chapter, we are going to explore the signs and symptoms that labor is on the way. You will also learn about some of the basic things that you should expect in the delivery room, and how you can prepare yourself for the experience.

Signs of Labor

The following symptoms are signs that labor is preparing to start. These symptoms are generally felt at some point between 37-40 weeks, if you carry your pregnancy all the way to term. However, you may experience these symptoms earlier than that if you are going into preterm labor. If you start experiencing any of these symptoms, especially before 37 weeks, you should consult your doctor. They will tell you what to do, and when you should come in!

Your Baby "Drops" Into Position

Before labor starts, your baby will "drop" into position. You can tell this has happened when your baby bump is sitting lower down, and is more directed towards your pelvis. This is because the baby has officially prepared to enter the birth canal, so they are getting lined up and ready to make an appearance!

Your Cervix Dilates

Probably the most well-known symptom of labor starting is the cervix dilating. Of course, you probably can't tell this is happening, but your doctor will be able to tell you. In the days leading up to your labor, your cervix will begin to slowly dilate. Most women sit around 1-2cm for about a week or two before labor actually begins. Once labor starts, they will continue opening until they reach 10cm, which is when active labor starts.

Increased Cramping and Lower Back Pain

You may notice more pain in your lower back and more cramping in your abdomen. This occurs as a result of your muscles preparing to put in all of the work to release your baby. This can also happen because the new position of your baby results in there being new pressures on your lower back and pelvic area. As well, your pelvis will be opening up the last little amount to let your baby come out, so your bones are quite literally stretching open.

LOOSER JOINTS

The increased progesterone in your system are still responsible for your joints being loose, though you may notice this even more towards labor. You may experience popping or cracking in your joints a lot more, particularly when you move out of a position you've been sitting in for the same amount of time for a while.

DIARRHEA

Many women experience diarrhea leading up to labor. This can be a displeasing opposite of the constipation that many women experience in the weeks beforehand. If you experience this, it's just because your muscles are loosening which means so are your bowel movements. Make sure you drink plenty of water, and prepare for labor to start!

YOUR WEIGHT GAIN SLOWS DOWN, OR YOU LOSE SOME WEIGHT

Once your baby is fully "cooked" they will pretty much stop putting on weight, because they are getting ready to come out! So, if you notice you've stopped putting on pounds, or even if you lose a couple, this is why!

YOU FEEL MORE FATIGUED THAN NORMAL

Because of your super-sized belly and all of your hormones, and the frequent need to urinate, it can be hard to get a full nights' rest. Because of this, you may find that you are consistently tired. The best thing you can do is sleep on the side closest to the washroom, and keep several pillows on hand to make those few hours of shut eye as restful as possible. As well, rest as much during the day as you can.

You Start Nesting

This is a common symptom of labor that you see often in the media on television shows and in movies. Nesting is a symptom many pregnant women experience towards the end of pregnancy as a means to prepare their home for the baby. If you find you suddenly have a burst of energy and all you want to do is clean and get everything ready for baby to come, it could be because baby is coming very soon!

Your Vaginal Discharge Changes

Changes in vaginal discharge can include increased or thickened discharge, and a change in color. This is completely normal.

Your Contractions Become Stronger and More Regular

As your Braxton Hicks contractions change to actual contractions, you may notice they become a lot stronger and more regular in frequency. This is your body preparing to contract the baby out, and unless they are happening minutes apart for a long period of time, it is completely normal.

BLOODY SHOW/MUCUS PLUG

As well as your vaginal discharge changing, you may experience your bloody show at some point. This happens as your mucus plug starts to fall out. You may notice a snot-like consistency that is streaked with blood. This is your mucus plug, and you don't need to worry about this, unless it's coming out before 37 weeks! Either way, you should tell this to your doctor just so they can be prepared for your impending labor!

YOUR WATER BREAKS

The water breaking is one of the most famously known labor symptoms, but also happens to be one of the ones that happen the least! Only about 15% of women experience this symptom, and it's usually the last sign that labor is about to start. Make sure you let your doctor know as soon as your water breaks, especially if it breaks early.

WHAT YOU SHOULD EXPECT IN THE DELIVERY ROOM

There are a lot of things to expect in the delivery room, and it varies based on how your pregnancy and labor have gone. If you are carrying a high-risk pregnancy, if you have a scheduled caesarean section, or if something goes wrong and your labor becomes an emergency caesarean section, you are going to have a totally different experience in the delivery room. In this chapter, we are going to only discuss what to expect in a healthy pregnancy where delivery occurs in a hospital room.

The delivery room is a scary and exciting place, and you may become overwhelmed with emotion while you are there. You are going to be going through a lot physically, and mentally. You are preparing to meet the life you've been creating for the past nine months, and that is a lot to take in! You are likely going to get hooked up to a no-stress-test machine that will make sure your fetal movements are strong and healthy, and to measure your contractions. You are also going to get your cervix checked on a fairly regular basis, to see how far you are progressing.

A good portion of your stay is going to be spent relaxing as much as possible so that you have the energy to get through the contractions. You may wish to spend some time in the shower or on a birthing ball, to help take some of the pressure and pain off of your abdomen. If it gets really hard, you may opt for pain medicines, such as laughing gas, or an epidural. If you were GBS positive, you will also be hooked up to an IV to get antibiotics every four hours.

Once labor begins, your doctor and a few nurses will come into the room. They will help coach you through pushing, and make sure your baby comes out safely. Your doctor may use forceps or a vacuum extractor to help take out your baby, if he or she needs a little assistance on the way out. Once your baby is out, your doctor will clamp the umbilical cord and let your partner cut the cord, if you have a partner involved. Then, you will be given a chance to have skin-to-skin contact with your baby, and nurse him or her. Sometime after your baby has been born, you will also have to push out your placenta, which is not a painful experience for most women, and takes minimal effort. The placenta is a tissue, so it will not stretch out your vagina as it exits your body, meaning you will likely not find it to be as painful, or painful at all.

Shortly after your baby is born, the nurses will take him or her for a few minutes to weigh your baby, and take some important measurements. You will then be able to shower off, and move into a more permanent room where you will remain for the rest of your hospital stay. About twenty-four hours after your baby is born, they will have their vitals taken to ensure that your baby is not suffering from jaundice or anything else. These are called heel-poke tests and they only take a few minutes for to do. Throughout the time you are there, your nurses will come in to check on you and your baby to ensure that you are both getting along well, and provide you with any support or assistance you may need along the way.

AN INSIGHT TO POSTPARTUM LIFE

The initial postpartum period is the hardest. You will be in "fourth trimester" until about six weeks after your baby is born. At this point, you are going to experience your postpartum bleeding, and many hormonal changes. Your body will be getting back into a balance from all of the pregnancy hormones, which can lead to many emotional and physical changes.

During these weeks, your baby is still going to have part of the umbilical cord - complete with the clamp - attached to their body. This will naturally fall off within' a few days once it dries up. Your baby may spit up a lot, which is completely normal as they are getting used to being able to digest food. Their poop is also weird, as it will be a blackish green color, or it could be yellow or brown. The color of newborn poop varies, and can also vary in texture. As long as it is not pale, you should be okay.

Getting to sleep through the night will be hard with your newborn, as they will want to eat frequently. Ideally, you should sleep during the day when your baby sleeps, at least for the first little while, as this will help you replenish the sleep you are losing through waking up all hours of the night. Having a strong support system in place is also helpful.

Chapter Six: Nutrition and Exercise During and After Pregnancy

Your nutrition and exercise during pregnancy and afterwards is important. You want to make sure you are maintaining your health, so that your baby stays healthy, too. In this chapter, you will learn exactly how you can do that, before and after pregnancy.

Nutrition

Eating healthy when you are pregnant is important. Many people will say you are "eating for two" now, and while you are, it can be hard to know exactly what that means. Luckily for you, we are going to explore exactly what you need to do to ensure that you are staying healthy enough to support yourself and your growing baby!

For food, you actually don't need to eat as much as you may think. In fact, if you have already been eating a healthy diet, your intake doesn't need to increase that much in the first trimester at all. The most important thing is to make sure that you are eating a healthy diet filled with fresh whole fruits and vegetables, grains, protein, calcium, and all of the regular important nutrition you'd regularly need! For your first trimester of pregnancy, you should try and eat the following each day:

- 3-4 servings of fresh fruits
- 3-5 servings of vegetables
- 3 servings of dairy
- 2-3 servings of protein
- 3 servings of whole grains

If you are struggling to eat this much each day, you can try alternative methods of ingesting foods, such as through juicing your fruits and vegetables or eating alternative forms of dairy that are easier to ingest. If you are still struggling, you can speak with your doctor to see if there are any methods you can use to increase your ability to get a healthy nutritional intake.

You are going to want to maintain these same intakes after pregnancy, particularly if you are nursing. Making sure you get adequate nutrients during the nursing time is important as it will help you continue to produce enough milk in order to feed your baby.

SUPPLEMENTS

The most important supplements for you to take during pregnancy are your Prenatal Vitamins and DHA supplements. These will help you keep your nutrient intake rich and strong, and ensure that you are getting adequate intake. The DHA is especially good for promoting healthy brain development in your fetus, among other benefits.

EXERCISE

When it comes to exercise in pregnancy, you want to make sure you are staying active, but you don't want to over-exert yourself. How much you should exercise will depend on your pre-pregnancy activity. If you were extremely active beforehand, you will be able to maintain a more active lifestyle. However, if you were not extremely active beforehand, or if you did not have a regular exercise routine, you will want to start implementing a light exercising routine into your daily activities. This can be hard if you are struggling from fatigue and morning sickness, so just make sure you are doing the best you can.

A great method of exercising and staying fit during pregnancy is through yoga. This activity is light and easy to do, and allows you to work at your comfort level without over exerting yourself. However, you should still avoid certain moves during yoga that could potentially cause damage to your ligaments. They are: backbends, any pose that requires you to twist your abdomen, positions where your feet go over your head, lying on your back (when you are further along in pregnancy) and hot yoga.

Other great ways to stay active include swimming, walking, and low-impact and low-intensity cardio. These allow you to stay active and keep moving without over exerting yourself or using an excessive amount of your energy. During the postpartum phase, you may wish to take up walking as a means to maintain a healthy activity level, without feeling the need to use extra energy you may not have during this time.

Chapter Seven: Tips for New and Expecting Fathers

As a Dad, you might feel many of the same emotions an expecting Mom would feel. You may be emotional, uncertain, excited, and worried. You may also feel added pressures of not knowing how to care for your pregnant wife and your newborn baby. In many cases, Dads are not provided with as much help during pregnancy, since it is the Mom who is carrying the pregnancy. However, it is just as important that you prepare yourself for the new baby as well. Here are some of the most common symptoms expectant fathers experience, and how you can manage them:

Feeling Left Out

With all of the emphasis on the Mom and the baby, it can be easy to feel left out during pregnancy and new parenthood. This is completely normal, and you should know that it won't always be this way. It may also be hard for you because you are not carrying the baby, therefore you are not experiencing all of the same developing connections as the Mom is. If you are feeling left out, you can try doing more to be involved. Spend time massaging your pregnant partner, speaking to the baby bump, and finding other ways to support your partner. Not only will she appreciate it, but it will help you feel better, too.

Feeling Disconnected

Particularly if you've been with your partner for a while before the baby was expected, you may feel a disconnection from your partner. Pregnancy will change things, causing your partner not to like what they used to love, and to like things you'd never dreamed they would. The best way to maintain the connection between you and your partner is to open the lines of communication.

Paternity Leave

Taking time off or getting paternity leave can be a tough spot for men. Many times, they want to be at home with their families, but don't know how to communicate this with their boss. It can certainly feel like an uncomfortable situation. The best thing to do is speak with your partner and ask for advice. Ideally, you should take at least a few days off to spend at home with your newborn and your wife who will be going through a number of hormonal and emotional changes at this time. If you can't, you should assist in ensuring she has a strong support team with her during this time.

Priorities Change

For some men, it can be hard to change their priorities when a baby is born. While a Mom has nine months to connect with the child and change her priorities, for men it can feel a lot more sudden. It can also be harder to let go of freedoms and have to become a family man, as you do not get the hormonal or instinctual changes that a woman will get. The best idea is to continue communicating with your partner and realize that your family is going to need you often, and that you are going to need to be present.

GETTING SUPPORT

Men need support just as much as women do, believe it or not. It is a good idea to get your support system in place, just as you are helping to do with your partner. This will allow you to have somewhere to turn if things are getting difficult. It can be hard to turn to your already stressed out partner at times, and though you should always be open with them, sometimes it can be helpful to also have backup support for when times get really hard.

If you are a Dad looking for more support or tips on how to handle pregnancy and postpartum, you can check out my other book: "Pregnancy: A Complete Guide for an Expectant Father".

Chapter Eight: Tips for Expecting Single Moms

Sometimes, there may not be a partner in the picture. If you are an expectant Mom who will also be a single Mom, it is equally as important that you prepare yourself and your new family for what is to come. There are many things you can do to help prepare yourself. Here are some of the best tips from other single Moms on how you can manage single parenthood.

Prepare for Your Emotions

Pregnancy and postpartum can bring a whirlwind of emotions and there is really no way around this. The best thing you can do is prepare for them. Have a game plan for what you will do when you are feeling particularly emotional, and execute it. The best game plans involve a lot of self-care, nurturing, and a solid support system.

Focus on Your Baby

When the baby is here, sometimes the best thing you can do when you are feeling overwhelmed is just focus on your baby. Pay attention to what they need and fulfill those needs. As long as your baby is cared for, you will have an easier time taking care of yourself, as well. When the baby is sleeping, that is when you can focus on taking care of your own needs, as well.

TAKE CARE OF BUSINESS

Single parents have to work a lot more than parents who have a partner, as unfortunate as that is. You should have a plan in place for how you will work, when you will return to work, and what you will do with your baby while you are working. If you are going to have daycare or babysitting, you should establish where your baby will go, well before you actually need to take them. If you are going to return to work soon after your baby, you should also have a plan as to what you will do if you are nursing, and how you will handle your emotions while on the job.

BUILD A SUPPORT TEAM

The most valuable thing a mother can have, especially as a single mother, is a strong support team. You should start building one during pregnancy. Your support team can include family, friends, online communities and professionals. Anyone who is capable of providing you with assistance is a valuable asset to your life and can help you greatly. In addition to building your support team, you should also make sure you reach out to them for help. If you need someone to come watch your baby while you get in extra sleep, ask for it. If you need help making some meals so you have food to eat during the day or the week, ask for it. Your support team is there to support you, so make sure you ask them.

THE CONCLUSION

Having a new baby is an exciting and stressful time for many. From all of the symptoms you will experience physically to all of the emotions you will experience that will mentally weigh on you, there is a lot you will go through. It is important that you brace yourself for everything that is to come.

Having this guidebook handy is a great way to recognize what symptoms are normal, and which are alarming. You can also prepare yourself for each trimester, and ensure that you are taking the best possible care of yourself. Even though pregnancy is a largely physical experience, you should also do your best to slow down and enjoy it. This may not be easy, especially if you are experiencing difficult symptoms or a high-risk pregnancy, but it is important since this experience is one you only get to have once in a lifetime.

It is important that you prepare yourself for childbirth well in advance, and that you maintain open lines of communication with everyone involved. The more open you are and honest you are about how you are feeling, the easier this process will be for you. Most importantly, stay calm and relaxed as much as possible, and nurture yourself in every way that you can to make this process as easy and as comfortable for you and your baby as possible.

www.ingramcontent.com/pod-product-compliance
Lightning Source LLC
Chambersburg PA
CBHW071245280526
45788CB00004B/1590